Intermittent Fasting - A Beginner's Guide to Quick Weight Loss

Introduction to Fasting for Dieting, Detoxing, Cleansing, Lifestyle, and Metabolism Boosts

By Sharon Kingsley

Aryla Publishing © 2019

www.arylapublishing.com
Visit the site for more information on books by Sharon Kingsley and to be informed of **free promotions!**

Please check out my other books

Giving Up Sugar

Diet Fads

The Christmas Diet

January Detox

Dieting Tips for a Healthier New You

Table of Contents

Introduction   7

Chapter 1: What is Intermittent Fasting?   10

Chapter 2: The Benefits of Intermittent Fasting   19

Chapter 3: How to Start   25

Chapter 4: Different Methods of Intermittent Fasting   31

How to Choose The Right Method For You   42

Chapter 5: Is Intermittent Fasting a Long-Term, Sustainable
Answer?   44

How Intermittent Fasting Can Help You Manage
Stress   46

Chapter 6: Sample Intermittent Fasting Menus   50

Chapter 7: Dos & Don'ts of Intermittent Fasting   62

Conclusion   72

Introduction

We're at that specific point of the year when everyone turns their attention towards weight loss. Whether you've decided to lose weight towards a healthier lifestyle, you want to lose weight to reach a goal, or you simply want to try and find a lifestyle which suits your needs better, you've come to the right place.

This book is about intermittent fasting.

The word 'fasting' tends to make people panic, and think that in some way they're going to be starving themselves. We all know that starving isn't healthy at all, so it's no wonder that this diet has a lot of mystery and misunderstanding surrounding it.

This book will bust those myths and show you that intermittent fasting can indeed be very healthy, when done the right way. There are countless ways to do intermittent fasting, e.g. many methods, and choosing the right one for you, to suit your lifestyle, will ensure that fasting fits in with your routine, and that you don't notice any adverse effects as a result.

Don't worry about the word 'fasting'. We've been fasting for millennia and it's actually ingrained in the way the human body words. As far back as the cavemen and cavewomen, who used to fast during times when food was lean, to save supplies for the future, humans have been fasting without adverse effects. There are many health benefits to be had from periods of fasting combined with periods of eating healthily, and one of them is certainly the fact that fasting does not give you the same unsuccessful dietary outcome as a regular or fad diet.

Intermittent fasting isn't a diet, it's a lifestyle choice. Intermittent dieting isn't a low calorie diet, because you're actually not restricting yourself to any type of food, you're just deciding when you can eat, versus when you are going to fast. Of course, that doesn't mean that during your 'able to eat' phase you can head to every fast food joint in town, but it does mean that if you want to have the odd treat, you can do so without feeling guilty and having to cut back on calories the next day. You do not need to account anything when you use intermittent fasting, you simply need to decide whether you're going to eat and when you're not.

There are bound to be countless questions about intermittent fasting in your mind, and you're probably a little concerned about not being able to eat. The thing is, we naturally fast every day - during our sleeping hours, usually around 7 to 8 hours everyday, we fast without even realising it! Does anything bad happen to us? No! Because we then have a period of eating which gives us the dietary nutrition we need. Intermittent fasting is the same basis, but with a few tweaks.

So, now we have explained what this book is about, it's time to delve into the world of intermittent fasting, and learn what it can bring to your life, as well as how to actually do it.

Chapter 1: What is Intermittent Fasting?

Having read the introduction to our book, you're now fully aware of what we're going to talk about. The fact you're still reading tells us that you're keen to learn more - great choice!

You might think that intermittent fasting is a new type of diet or lifestyle choice, but it's actually been around for countless years. Humans naturally fast during certain times in their life, either because food is scarce (as per the caveman example we gave earlier), or due to religious reasons, e.g. during the Muslim Holy month of Ramadan, when Muslims fast between sunrise and sunset.

When done correctly, intermittent fasting can bring a whole host of benefits to your life, and we're going to explore those in more detail in our next chapter. For now, you simply need to know that by adopting an intermittent fasting lifestyle, you're handing control over your health and weight to yourself and yourself alone. You don't have to count calories, you don't have to force your body into any type of metabolic state, and you don't need to push yourself to remember macros and ratios. You simply need to eat when you can and not when you can't. In-between those times you can drink water and unsweetened black tea or black coffee. It's that simple!

You've no doubt got many questions, so let's start with the most basic of them all - how exactly does this all work?

How Does Fasting Work?

Intermittent fasting is the process of eating for a set number of hours per day, and then fasting for the rest. You can mix up your times of eating versus not eating according to several different methods, and we'll talk about those in far more detail in a later chapter.

The idea is that you are giving your body a regular and sustainable amount of nutrition, but you are also having a break, which allows your body to use up that nutrition and therefore not binge, or go over what it needs. Ironically, intermittent fasting means that you are giving your body a regular and constant source of calories, but within a normal bracket. Most of us consume far too many calories during a regular day, because we can eat whenever we want. This is the single reason for weight gain.

The reason you will lose weight on the intermittent fasting lifestyle is that you are actually consuming less calories and you are probably also pushing your body to start burning fat as an energy source also, depending upon the method you choose. This obviously gives you weight loss because you're eating into those fat reserves that you detest so much (probably). You also don't need to be a scientist to realise that if you eat less calories than you burn, you lose weight!

The reason that people choose intermittent fasting over regular low calorie diets is that there is no huge amount of restriction. You can eat a chocolate bar if you want to, when you're permitted to eat, and it won't ruin your entire dieting day. If you're on a low calorie diet, that chocolate bar is probably going to take up a huge portion of the calories you're allowed to consume in that day!

Of course, you still need to eat healthily in order to notice weight loss, otherwise you're probably just going to stick at your current weight or even put weight on, but if you are careful with your food choices and throw in some exercise for good measure, intermittent fasting is a fantastic way to lose weight and gain health benefits, with very little in the way of effort.

Surely that's what we all want!

Is Intermittent Fasting Safe and Sustainable?

Intermittent fasting is perfectly safe as long as you do it correctly, i.e. you eat when you are supposed to and you stay hydrated throughout the entire day, by drinking water and unsweetened tea and coffee (black tea and black coffee). You shouldn't consume any calories during the fasting period, but during your eating period, that's when you need to abide by the rules and eat sensibly and well.

If you overload your stomach with far too much high fat food, simply because you can eat for those few hours, you're going to a) probably put weight on, and b) overload your stomach to the point where you experience discomfort. You'll learn that you feel far better when you eat healthily within your fasting routine, and that will be enough to keep you going.

We've talked already about the fact that humans have been fasting for years, and it's perfectly healthy, in fact in some cases it can be encouraged. For instance, if you've been ill, a doctor might advise you to fast for a few hours in order to detox your body and cleanse your stomach, before you begin to eat light meals and build yourself up to eating normally again. There is a huge difference between fasting and starving.

Is it sustainable. Very. There are so many different methods of intermittent fasting that it's easy to choose one which really fits in with your lifestyle. That way, you're not really making any sacrifices, and it will simply become just another part of your daily routine. You don't need to count anything, weight anything out, or become super-au fait with food labels. You simply need to know when to eat and when not to, and make sensible choices in general. It's so easy!

Differences Between Fasting And Starving

The reason that intermittent fasting has got a slightly bad reputation is nothing to do with the way it works or whether it's safe or not, and it's entirely down to the word 'fasting' which is in the title! We misinterpret the word 'fasting' and confuse it with 'starving'.

Starving yourself is totally different to fasting. When you're fasting, you're not choosing not to eat, you're simply having a break from it. When you're starving yourself, you're signalling the intention to not eat, which will have detrimental effects on your health and wellbeing. In many cases, starvation is fatal. Fasting is not.

A person who is starving, either intentionally or unintentionally, will not have periods of eating versus periods of not eating - they simply won't eat at all. They might drink water in order to stay hydrated, but food will not pass their lips. A person with anorexia, for example, is not fasting, they are starving themselves. That is what makes eating disorders so dangerous. Do not confuse fasting with conditions such as this, because when you are choosing to fast, you are making a healthy decision, provided you follow the rules. When you choose to starve yourself, you're basically signing your own death certificate.

Who Shouldn't Fast?

There is no eating routine or lifestyle which is suitable for every single person on the planet, and the same can be said for intermittent fasting. It actually comes down to the type of routine you choose, i.e. the method of intermittent fasting, in many ways. There are only a few people who aren't suitable for fasting, because it's a natural part of life for centuries. There are however some anomalies. The following people shouldn't follow an intermittent fasting lifestyle:

• Pregnant women
• Anyone with a serious health condition

For everyone else, it's about speaking to your doctor and finding out a medical opinion on whether this lifestyle is for you. From there, it's equally about doing your research into the specific methods of intermittent fasting, and then choosing the one which will give you nutritious value when you need it. Luckily for you, we're going to talk in more detail about specific methods a little later on. Equally, if you start to feel unwell whilst you're following an intermittent fasting method, it could simply be that you have chosen the wrong routine for you, and you need to think again.

Fasting For Religious Reasons

The most famous incidence of fasting for a religious reason is during the Muslim Holy month of Ramadan. During this month, Muslims who choose to observe Ramadan do not eat between the hours of sunrise and sunset. When the sun has gone down, they eat healthy and light foods, to avoid overloading their stomach.

Ramadan teaches Muslims about value of things in life though the sacrifice of not eating during these specific times, and as a result of the fasting, many people say that they feel more enlightened, closer to God, more focused, and have greater value for everything and everyone in their lives. This is a common benefit which is often mentioned when fasting of any kind is raised.

Islam is not the only religion which has links with fasting, as in Christianity, the period of Lent also connects with fasting. Whilst people tend to give up something which is important to them at this time, some fast instead. The Jewish faith also includes fasting as part of Yom Kippur, and Hinduism also has links with fasting.

As you can see, fasting for religious reasons is nothing new, and is certainly not only confined to Islam. The idea is that you are closer to God and more enlightened as a result of the detox your body is going through, whilst teaching you important lessons mentally. Fasting is a sacrifice in this context, but is done safely with periods of eating versus periods of fasting.

Fasting For Cleansing

Many detoxes include fasting as a way of cleaning out the body of impurities and toxins. This includes a period of not eating (fasting), versus a period of eating only specific types of foods, e.g. extremely nutritious and antioxidant packed foods, which bring goodness and cellular regeneration to the body.

Cleaning routines have been around for many years, and there are also health retreats which offer fasting programmes for detoxing.

Fasting in general allows the body to naturally remove waste products, i.e. toxins which clog up the body and cause it to run sluggishly and slowly. By eliminating toxins, you feel lighter, more energised, see improvement in skin and also in concentration.

In these routines, fasting tends to be a day or two day long process, and doesn't have the eating and then fasting routine which many intermittent fasting methods do.

Fasting in Protest

Finally we have fasting for a protesting reason. There is a difference between fasting for cleaning and religious reasons and fasting in protest. Many people who are fasting as a protest are actually starving themselves in some way. They don't want to take it all the way, but they are, in effect, threatening that they will starve to death for their cause. You will have heard the phrase 'hunger strike' and that is basically what we're talking about here.

Fasting for a protest isn't really something to consider and is very dangerous and unhealthy. In this case, a protestor will normally eat liquid foods, but will refuse solids. The idea is that you are causing the person you're protesting against, or the system, to feel guilty and therefore bring about a change in policy, or in whatever you're protesting against.

This type of fasting is not going a process of eating for a short while and then not eating for a short while, and is more likely to be a longer period of simply not eating at all. The fact that this type of fasting is unhealthy is the reason why those on hunger strike do it - they are attempting to shock or bring feelings of guilt to those they're protesting against.

By this point in the book you should be quite clear on the fact that intermittent fasting isn't dangerous, and isn't anything like starving. The ironic thing about fasting is that you won't feel hungry after a while. Your body will fall into routine and you won't have those cravings and hunger pangs associated with other diets, because your body is not being deprived of anything per se, e.g. you aren't avoiding eating a specific food because it's high in calories, you're simply eating in a different way, at a different time. You're allowing your body to fall into a pattern which it will anticipate and learn how to adapt to quite quickly.

Don't worry if you still have a lot of questions about intermittent fasting, that's normal. We're talking about a very big change in your lifestyle here, and having more questions is very common. In our next chapter, we're going to talk about the benefits of adopting an intermittent fasting lifestyle.

Chapter 2: The Benefits of Intermittent Fasting

You might wonder how fasting can actually bring any benefits to your body, but be prepared to be astounded! Intermittent fasting has many beneficial effects for the mind and body overall, provided you follow the rules and eat during the times you're supposed to eat.

The main benefits of intermittent fasting include:

- **Weight loss and loss of body fat** - This is down to the fact that in general you are eating less calories throughout the whole day without even realising it. You are also more likely to lose fat pockets, because your body is using up fat to burn as energy also.
- **Higher levels of concentration and clarity** - When your body is purified of toxins, and you're cleansed from the inside out, your mind will be far sharper. Many people who following fasting lifestyles mention their mental clarity as the first benefit. Of course, weight loss is the most common reason that people fast, but the ability to think more clearly and make better decisions overall is a fantastic plus point to think about.
- **Blood sugar levels are regulated and type II diabetes may be reduced** - Because you're spreading out a lower calorie intake over a longer period of time, you're forcing your body to work in a different way. The main benefit of this is lower blood sugar levels and also lower insulin levels. For anyone who suffers from type II diabetes, this has major potential to improve the condition, and in some cases, possibly even reverse it.
- **Far more energy** - Once again, this is down to the cleansing process which detoxes the body of impurities. Many of these toxins and impurities cause

sluggishness, not only in the body but also in the brain. When you feel free of these toxins, you are more energised in general, and you feel lighter on your feet and in your mind. The energising effect of intermittent fasting is a great benefit to obtain.

- **Inflammation reduction** - Inflammation is responsible for a huge number of different conditions and problems within the body. When inflammation markers are high, the body reacts in many negative ways. For instance, someone with arthritis has generally high inflammatory markers, causing pain and stiffness. Inflammation is also the body's natural method of protecting itself, e.g. when you sprain your ankle, you see inflammation as a way of protecting the injury. Intermittent fasting helps to reduce general inflammatory markers, which can help to reduce many problems and decrease the effects of certain conditions.
- **Cell generation via a process called autophagy** - During fasting, the body may use a process called autophagy. This is when the body basically consumes itself, but it isn't as bad as it sounds! This is a cleansing and detoxing process which removes old and dead cells and helps to boost the growth and production of new ones. Autophagy in itself has many benefits, including improved skin conditions and more energy overall.
- **Better sleep quality** - Nothing cravings, not being hungry, and basically feeling healthier and more at ease has a fantastic effect on your sleep pattern and quality of sleep overall. When you have a quality sleep pattern, everything falls into place and you'll feel more able to take on the world as a result.
- **Lower cholesterol levels** - Through eating a heather diet and consuming less calories (from high fat foods), your cholesterol levels are naturally lowered. Fasting is also linked with lower cholesterol. We all know that

high cholesterol levels are dangerous for overall health and wellbeing and can increase the risk of heart attack and stroke.

- **The potential to live longer** - Whilst there aren't any specific studies which can prove this either way for sure, the fact that you are healthier overall, with less risk factors for serious disease, means that you are likely to live longer. You will hear people shouting about longer lives with fasting, but this isn't something you can bank on - none of us know about that! What you can bank on is the accumulation of the other benefits which could elongate your life due to better health overall.

The biggest non-health benefit is about ease. Intermittent fasting doesn't cause the complications which other diets do. You don't need to count things, you don't need to eat specific foods and cut others out completely, in fact you don't need to limit yourself at all.

Intermittent fasting is a very easy to follow and simple way of life, and it is also a less expensive option too. When you compare this method with others, like the Keto Diet, you don't have to buy anything special to follow it. Whilst it's obviously better to opt for organic and fresh produce whenever possible, you don't have to make such firm decisions when you follow the fasting way of life. You can be more flexible, and this can save you cash as well as stress. Fasting also easily fits around your lifestyle, i.e. work and home. You can find a method which allows you to eat at the times you need it, and then fast at the times you can manage without.

Possible Side Effects of Intermittent Fasting

Are there any downsides?

There's always a downside to everything in some way, and intermittent fasting is no different. This won't suit everyone, and perhaps you try it and realise that it's not for you. If that's the case, that's fine, you tried it out, but the likelihood is that you simply need to tweak a few things and it will work better for you from that point onwards.

The side effects which occur should pass quite quickly, after your body has transitioned and got used to the routine you've put into place. The most common side effects are:

- **Hunger at first** - When your body has got used to eating at specific times throughout the day, it's common to experience hunger when you first start changing the entire pattern. This will pass once your body gets used to your new routine, but at first, you might notice that during the times you're fasting, you're quite hungry. What you will come to realise also is that a lot of the time when you think you're hungry, you're actually bored or thirsty instead. Try and distract yourself by doing something, going for a walk, having a drink of water, or having a relaxing bath instead.
- **Cravings** - The same can be said for cravings. The cravings you may experience at first with intermittent dieting are not going to be anywhere near as bad as diets which restrict your calorie intake to low amounts and tell you that you can't eat x, y, and z ever again. What you're experiencing at first is that transitional

period, which will pass when your body once again gets used to what is happening. After that, you shouldn't have cravings because, within reason, you can eat what you want during your eating times.

- **Headaches** - In the first week or so, you might notice an increase in headaches, but provided these aren't too severe, you can be reassured that they are simply a side effect of your body transitioning once more. This can also be because your blood sugar levels are reducing and your body isn't used to it yet, as well as stress. The fact your body is getting used to eating at different times can actually cause stress that you're not aware of. Relax as much as possible and drink water, and they should pass relatively quickly.
- **Lacking energy** - Again, once you start to get into the full swing of intermittent fasting, you'll quickly realise that your energy levels are on the rise, but at first, this might not be the case. Rest up and eat foods during your eating phase which are slow release, to give you a boost of energy during your fasting times.
- **Feeling annoyed or irritated** - This links to hunger and cravings, because we all feel that way when we're hungry. The phase 'hangry' was made for a reason - you're hungry and angry because you want to eat! Again, this is your body not really understanding quite yet what is going on, but once it figures it all out, the problem should go away.

These are the most common side effects, so if you're noticing these, you're in the majority. Remember, we're all different so it could be that you have a different side effect, or you might not have any at all. The best thing to do is to monitor any affects you have and simply be mindful of how you feel. If you notice anything untoward or you simply don't feel right, speak to your doctor and try and work out which intermittent fasting method is better suited to you, if any at all.

Chapter 3: How to Start

Now you know what intermittent fasting is, and you know why it is a good option for you, as well as the possible transitional period side effects, it's time to get practical!

In our next chapter, we're going to talk in far more detail about the different types of intermittent fasting and how to make them work, e.g. when you can eat versus when you need to fast. For that reason, when you're checking out the steps we're about to mention, you need to factor in the specifics of your chosen fasting method too.

Overall however, we can talk generally about how to begin with any intermittent fasting method.

Step 1 - Signal Your Intention And Reason Why

The first step is to decide that you want to try intermittent fasting in general and the reason you want to try it. Having the reason in your mind, rather than being vague, means that you can be more specific. If you have a moment of not being sure why you're doing this, e.g. in the beginning when you might notice the odd side effect, having the reason in your mind will get you through that 'wobble' and keep you going. So, make a pledge to yourself that you're going to make intermittent fasting work for you, and write down the specific reason on why you have chosen it, and why you want to do it. Whenever you're not sure anymore, or you're struggling, look at that piece of paper.

Step 2 - Speak to Your Doctor

Now you have decided that you want to try it and you know why, it's time to get the green light from your doctor. Check that you do not have any contraindications to fasting overall, e.g. you're not pregnant, and have a chat with your doctor. Tell him or her that you want to try intermittent fasting and ask for their opinion, taking into account any conditions you have or medications you're on. Make sure that you listen to their advice and take it on board. Never go against medical advice, purely because you want fast weight loss - it's really not worth the detrimental effects that could come your way, and instead you would be better searching for a different option.

For most people however, intermittent fasting won't be contraindicated and provided your doctor gives you the go ahead, you can move onto the next step in your starting process.

Step 3 - Educate Yourself on The Different Fasting Methods

Now you need to sit down and read. In our next chapter, we're going to talk about the different intermittent fasting methods you can try and how they work. From there, you can identify which one might be best for you, and perhaps do some deeper research if you feel you need to. Being armed with as much information as possible is the single best way to make an informed, quality decision overall.

Step 4 - Choose Your Fasting Method

Having done your homework on the main types of intermittent fasting, you can now make your choice.

Remember, if you make a choice and you find it's just not working that well for you, you can always go back and try a different one. This isn't a set in stone or concrete choice!

Find the method which fits in with your lifestyle, e.g. if you work part time, full time, if you work evenings, whether you have a family, or if you have hobbies which you want to do at certain times. There is a method which will suit every type of routine, and it's just a case of being a little flexible and identifying the ideal choice.

Once you've made your decision, write down the guidelines, e.g. the times when you can eat versus the times when you're fasting. Keep this together with the piece of paper about your reason for wanting to do this whole thing in the first place. When you're not sure or you're confused about what you should be doing at that moment, you can do a quick reference and you're back in control.

Step 5 - Declutter Your Kitchen of Temptation

The next step is to declutter and get rid of any temptation! There are two reasons for this step. Firstly, when you first start to fast, you're going to experience a little hunger and some cravings. That could lead you to giving into temptation and ruining your fast before you even get into the swing of it. By throwing out all temptation, you can side step that issue and take back control.

The other side is that even though you aren't limited with what you can and can't eat during your eating phases, you do need to keep health at the forefront of your mind. It's not a good idea to eat cookies, pizzas, and burgers during your eating phase, because you're going to consume a day's worth of calories in one meal, and you're also going to overload your stomach with heavy, high fat foods, which will leave you with a stomach ache and possibly some other rather unpleasant effects. Go shopping and pack your fridge and cupboards with healthy foods which you are going to enjoy, and then allow yourself the odd treat here and there. That's the best way to manage your eating phases healthily.

Step 6 - Take it One Day at a Time

Now you're ready to start on your first day! Do not think ahead and do not rush. Work one day at a time and with every day that passes, you'll feel the possible side effects of the transitional period wearing off, and you'll start to feel wonderful in yourself. Take it slowly and avoid stressing yourself out in the first few days.

It is a good job however to keep a journal, because that way you'll be able to identify your progress, but you'll also be able to spot any adverse effects that might be building up.

Step 7 - Review Your Method After The First Week

Once the first week is out of the way, firstly, pat yourself on the back and congratulate yourself! Secondly, it's time to sit down and review whether you've chosen the right intermittent fasting method, or whether you think after a week of experience you should have gone with a different option. Look at your journal at this point, as that will help to bring information to your mind that you might have otherwise forgotten.

If you are happy with your current method, that's fine, just continue onwards. If you think you might like to change it up, start the following day. Do bear in mind however, if you change your method of fasting, you may extend the amount of time that you experience side effects, because your body will need more time to adjust. It will be worth it in the end however, when you find the ideal method that suits your mind, body, and your lifestyle well.

Step 8 - Continue or Tweak

Now all that's left to do is to continue onwards with your chosen method or tweak it, as we mentioned before. Keep writing that journal to be able to identify any issues more clearly, and keep reviewing as you go along, perhaps on a monthly basis from that point onwards.

As you can see, beginning your intermittent fasting journey doesn't have to be a major drama, and it can be quite an easy process, provided you don't try and run before you can walk. Take it step by step and know that you can alter your method at any time, if you think it isn't suiting you as well as you first thought.

Chapter 4: Different Methods of Intermittent Fasting

There are many different types of intermittent fasting methods around, and it really comes down to choosing the ideal one for your needs. Read each description carefully and try and imagine how it would work for you. Remember, if you choose a method and you find it's not the ideal one, you can always change at a later date - your decision is not set in stone!

Let's explore each one of the most common methods in turn.

5:2 Diet

You will find the 5:2 Diet also called the Fast Diet, and it is the most popular of all the intermittent fasting methods. The name comes from the method of eating, e.g. you will eat normally for five days of the week, with a healthy and varied diet, and then you will limit your calories quite drastically for the other two days, eating no more than 500-600 calories during those two days.

The plus point of this particular diet is that you don't need to actually fast, e.g. have periods where you can't eat. The two 'fasting' days are actually very low calorie days, but it is important to make sure that you get the 500-600 calories during those days, for your overall health and wellbeing. During the rest of the week, you'll be able to eat freely, but make sure that you make healthy choices, and that you don't go all out eating whatever you want. In that case, you'll gain weight instead.

Despite that, the days when you can eat freely do not restrict anything, it's simply up to you to figure out what healthy is for you. This diet is therefore very easy to stick to and more of a way of life than an actual diet. For that reason, many people really like this method and find it super-easy to follow, no matter what their lifestyle.

The rules of this diet are:

- You will eat normally for five days of the week, out of seven
- During these five days, you do not have to restrict your calories, but you should try and eat healthy, for overall wellbeing
- You will then reduce your calorie intake down to 500 if you're a woman, and 600 if you're a man, for two days of the week
- The five days of eating and two days of restriction can be any days you like, but the limited days need to have a 'normal' day between them, i.e. don't have the two limited days together. A common option is to have your calorie limited days on Tuesdays and Fridays, with the rest of the days unlimited, but the choice is yours

Pros of The 5:2 Diet

- You don't actually have to fast, e.g. there are no specific hours when you don't eat at all
- You have control over what you eat for five days of the week
- You can make your lower calorie days easier by eating two small meals and deferring breakfast until later in the day

- You will lose weight quite quickly provided you don't over-indulge during your regular five days of eating
- This diet is good for building lean muscle
- It is very easy to follow and fits in with most lifestyles

Cons of The 5:2 Diet

- You have to be wary of not eating too much of the wrong kind of things during the five days you can eat freely
- 500 - 600 calories (depending on your gender) is a low amount and during these days you're likely to experience hunger and cravings
- Your low-calorie days might not be the most enjoyable, but you need to find ways to distract your mind and eat foods which are extremely low in calories, but still delicious

16:8 Diet

The 16:8 Diet is a popular choice of intermittent fasting methods. Basically, with this eating pattern you eat normally for 8 hours of the day, and you fast for the other 16. Now, 16 hours sounds like a long time to fast for, but you are probably going to be sleeping for 8 of those hours, which makes it much easier to handle!

You can choose to follow this eating pattern every day, or you can limit it to a couple of times per week, it's entirely up to you and what you're trying to achieve. If weight loss is your goal then having a daily routine is probably best, and will also limit hunger pang side effects on the days when you are fasting for those 16 hours.

The rules of the 16:8 Diet are:

- You choose a window of 8 consecutive hours during the day when you will eat normally
- During these 8 hours, you need to eat healthily, but you are not restricted. Remember, binging during these hours will not bring you health benefits or weight loss
- You then need to fast for the remaining 16 hours of the day. This can include your sleeping hours
- A good example is to choose to eat from 12pm until 8pm, and then fast until the following midday. For some people this works well because they can't stomach breakfast when they first wake up

The plus point of this particular eating pattern, rather than the one we just talked about is that you don't have to limit your calories on any day, it's more about just not eating for specific hours. Those hours can be cut down into sleeping and waking hours, and provided you eat foods which are slow release and leave you with enough energy until bedtime when sleep takes over, you really shouldn't notice a difference. During your fasting hours, you are able to drink water, and calorie-free drinks, such as black, unsweetened tea or coffee. This should be enough in the morning for a caffeine fix until your eating hours can begin.

Pros of The 16:8 Diet

- The 16:8 Diet is extremely easy to follow once you have chosen your eating and fasting times

- The fasting time can also include your sleeping hours, which cuts down on the waking times you might be hungry otherwise
- This pattern of eating fits in well with most lifestyles and gives you total control over what you eat and when
- You don't have any limitations on your calorie intake during the hours you can eat, however you shouldn't binge on unhealthy options, because that will simply lead to you eating more calories overall

Cons of The 16:8 Diet

- During the fasting hours, you might experience hunger if you choose the wrong window. This is something you can alter if it doesn't work well for you
- If you choose to have a late breakfast, you might experience low energy in the mornings
- There is a risk of eating too much during the 'eating hours', which leads to extra calories and also to stomach aches due to overloading the stomach

800 Fast Diet

The 800 Fast Diet is one of the newest around and was created by Dr Michael Mosley. You'll find many books on this diet at the moment, as it is the newest kid on the block. Basically, the 800 Fast Diet is a combination of a fasting and low calorie option, and it has two phases.

- During the first two weeks, you will consume 800 calories per day
- After those two weeks, you then revert to the 5:2 Diet, which we described above, but with a few changes

- The new version of the 5:2 Diet as the second phase means you eat freely during five days the week, with two days of consuming 800 calories per day. On those low-calorie days, you must eat your meals within a window 10 hours, and no later. This method is called time restricted feeding

Basically, you're getting drastic weight loss in the first two weeks, but you can't remain on that any longer than this time, because it's simply not sustainable or healthy. So, after the two weeks have elapsed, you will then move onto the easier to follow 5:2, giving you ease of eating what you like (within reason) during five days of the week, with two days of the regular 800 calories you were used to before. The only difference is that on those low-calorie days the 10-hour window comes into effect. The idea behind this is that you are forcing your body to burn fat rather than calories, therefore continuing your weight loss and health benefits.

The 800 Fast Diet, being the new kid on the block, is understandably the most popular at the moment, and once those restrictive two weeks are over, the maintenance phase (the newer 5:2 version) is easy to continue with long-term.

Pros of The 800 Fast Diet

- During the first two weeks of restricted calories you will lose quite a lot of weight quickly
- After the two weeks, you can eat more of what you like, following the regular 5:2 Diet, but with the higher amount allowed on the other two days (800 calories), and within a 10-hour window. You will then fast for the remaining hours, until the next day

- This is an easy to follow diet, once the first two weeks are over
- High amounts of weight loss in the first two weeks, which will slow down but still continue after that
- You do not need to restrict your calories in the second stage, for five days of the week

Cons of The 800 Fast Diet

- The first two weeks will be difficult, due to the low-calorie intake you are allowed
- You have to consume your meals during 10 hours when you reach the second stage and you are on your two days of limited calories
- There is little more complication in terms of when you can do what with this diet, but you should fall into a pattern relatively quickly
- Once you finish your two weeks of low calories, it might be very easy to binge on unhealthy options, because you've missed eating certain things

Warrior Diet

The intermittent fasting methods we've talked about so far have been quite easy to understand and follow and apart from the two weeks of low calorie intake on the Fast Diet, not so difficult in terms of cravings or hunger. The Warrior Diet really stands out from the rest of the diets we've talked about because it has longer phases of fasting and actually encourages overeating during a short window in the night.

The Warrior Diet was designed by a member of the Special Forces of Israel in 2001, and utilises the body's survival techniques, e.g. how it survives when it thinks there is no food. Of course, there is food, and you're not going to starve, but you are kick-starting the body's natural defenses and using them for your own greater good. The name comes from the warriors of ancient times, who used to eat very little throughout daylight hours, but then feasted to their heart's content during the night.

The rules of the Warrior Diet include:

- You do not eat for 20 hours of the day, but you eat whatever and as much as you like at night time, for the remaining 4 hours of the 24-hour span of time
- During the 20 hours of fasting, you aren't fasting per se, as you can eat very small amounts of dairy, including eggs which are hard boiled, raw vegetables and fresh raw fruits. You should also make sure that you drink plenty of fluids, which have no calories, such as water or unsweetened black tea or coffee
- During the remaining 4 hours, you can eat whatever you like, however many calories it contains

The problem with the Warrior Diet is that you are in effect binge eating during the 4-hour window, and that means you're certainly going to choose very high fat options. Firstly, you need the fat content because you haven't had any throughout the day, but you're also likely to be overloading your stomach. This will almost certainly lead to stomach disturbances of some kind, at least at first. Despite that, the Warrior Diet does bring weight loss and a few other health benefits.

Pros of The Warrior Diet

- Guaranteed weight loss, which is quite likely to be large
- You can eat all your favourite foods without restriction during the 4-hour eating window
- There are certain foods you can eat during the fasting period, so you're not fasting in the strictest sense

Cons of The Warrior Diet

- Not eating properly for 20 hours is going to make you hungry and as a result you're certainly going to binge on unhealthy options when you are allowed to eat
- Binge eating isn't particularly healthy in general, and stomach upsets are likely
- You'll need a lot of will power for this one!

Alternate Day Fasting

As the name would suggest, alternate day fasting means that you fast one day and eat what you want the next. This means you never have to miss out on what you want, but you do need to kind of pay for it the next day! There are modified versions of this type of intermittent fasting route, which may make the fasting times easier also.

The idea behind this type of method is that you're only really giving yourself any type of restriction for half the time and then you can eat whatever you want - within reason. The modified version means that on the fasting day, you can actually consume 500 calories, so you would have a normal eating day, followed by a 500-calorie day, followed by normal eating day, and so on.

The rules of the alternate day fasting method are:

- You eat normally on one day, having whatever you want within reason
- The following day you fast and eat nothing, except for drinking water, and unsweetened and black tea and coffee
- The next day you eat normally and then fast the following day
- The other option is that you eat normally one day and then eat a limited number of calories the next day (500) and then follow the same pattern as above

Many people find this method much easier to stick to, but the fasting days can be hard going. For that reason, if you find the complete fasting days too difficult, the modified version is something you can give a go.

Pros of Alternate Day Fasting

- You can eat freely during the alternate 'eating' days, which means you don't have to give anything up
- You can choose whether to fast on the other days, or have a low number of calories, at 500
- You will lose weight with this method, whilst still being able to have what you want
- You can also continue with your regular lifestyle, e.g. going out for meals with friends etc, you simply need to make sure these events fall on your eating days
- Very easy to follow and no need to count hours or anything else

Cons of Alternate Day Fasting

- The fasting days might be very hard, especially at first
- If you opt for 500 calories on the fasting days, this is still a very low amount and is likely to cause hunger, cravings, and irritability. Thankfully, you can eat the next day!
- At first, you're likely to binge a little on the eating days, because the fasting days will be difficult when you first begin

How to Choose The Right Method For You

We've spoken about the main types of intermittent fasting routines, and there are sure to be many more cropping up in the near future, as this type of eating pattern becomes even more popular. Finding the method which fits your needs is vital, if you want to make intermittent fasting a sustainable part of your life. The questions you need to ask yourself about each method before making your choice are:

- Is this method sustainable for me?
- Does it fit in with my lifestyle and will it stop me doing any of the things I enjoy?
- Will I be able to do the fasting periods, e.g. however long they are?
- Does this method make sense to me?

Those questions should help you make your choice, but remember, if you feel you've made the wrong decision, you can always go back and change it in the future.

The method you choose has to make sense to you because if you can't understand it or really get to grips with how and why it works, how are you supposed to follow it properly? We mentioned during the section on how to begin with fasting, that you need to know why you're going to try intermittent fasting in the first place. If you don't signal your intention and understand your reason, when times get a little tough, you'll give up before the benefits even have chance to start. The same line of thought should be adopted in choosing the right eating pattern. Choose the one which makes the most sense for you, not anybody else.

Chapter 5: Is Intermittent Fasting a Long-Term, Sustainable Answer?

We've talked in detail about the specific fasting methods and we've shown you what a typical day will look like on each one. This should help you choose the right option for you, but again, you need to think carefully before you make your decision. What we need to explore now is whether or not intermittent fasting is really a long-term, sustainable answer for life.

Fad diets come and go, and we all know that low calorie diets really aren't much fun in the long term. How many of you have tried a calorie restricted diet and actually stuck to it for a long-term period of time? You probably managed it for a short time, but then gave up because, let's face it, life's too short to not eat the things you love! Food is designed to be enjoyed and whilst we eat for nutrition, we also eat within a sociable element too. Food is at the heart of everything. For instance, we eat dinner with family, we meet friends for food, we have snacks when watching a movie at the cinema with someone special, we grab coffee and cake when we're catching up with someone we haven't seen in a long time. Food features in most events.

That isn't because we place it there, it's because food is a natural backdrop to a social time. We eat and we drink because that is what humans do, and why shouldn't we enjoy delicious food? There are so many amazing and healthy recipes out there which not only nourish our bodies, but also treat our taste buds, so why are we denying ourselves the pleasure?

The great thing about the intermittent fasting lifestyle is that you're not denying yourself a single thing, and whilst there are some routines which are a little more restrictive, you have the power to make your own food-related decisions. For instance, if you follow the 5:2 Diet, you can easily still go out for dinner with friends, go to a party, go to the cinema and enjoy snacks, you simply make sure that you arrange it to happen on one of the five days you can eat normally. There is no restriction there, because you're eating normally for the vast majority of the time!

The Warrior Diet is without a doubt the most restrictive all the intermittent fasting methods we've covered, and that is probably only going to be for someone who wants seriously fast and quite drastic results. Is it sustainable? If you have a lot of will power yes, but for most people, no. Whilst this is still popular option to choose from, mainly because of the results it promises, it isn't the one that most people go for first of all.

The Fast Diet is a middle ground choice. There is a period of two weeks which are quite hard going, but after that you're basically eating quite normally, apart from a lower calorie two days of the week. These two days are higher in calorie content than the restricted days on the 5:2 Diet, which gives you more leeway in what you can eat and enjoy during those two 'fasting' days.

Really, intermittent fasting methods aren't the regular type of fasting. You're not denying yourself for very long periods of time, and if you arrange your fasting windows correctly, you can cut down how much it will affect you, because you'll be sleeping. When you're fast asleep, you're not concerning yourself with hunger or food cravings, which makes it a win-win!

So, is intermittent fasting sustainable? If you choose the right method, yes, it is. This is a far more simplistic and successful diet than a low-calorie option, and far less stressful than choosing something like the Atkins or Keto Diet, which means you need to count and be careful of carb intake, so as not to throw your body's natural ketosis state out of whack. If you've followed the Keto Diet for any length of time, or even read about it, you'll understand that whilst it's a very do-able way of life and it has some great choices in terms of recipes, it's not the easiest to follow in terms of social events. Intermittent fasting doesn't impact on your lifestyle in any way, shape, or form, provided you choose the right method.

How Intermittent Fasting Can Help You Manage Stress

One of the biggest problems of the modern day is stress. We are always running around trying to finish one task, whilst in the middle of another. In a lot of ways, stress is actually responsible for poor health and weight gain.

When our bodies are in the midst of a stress response, a hormone called cortisol is released. This is more commonly known as the 'stress hormone'. It's normal to have a certain amount of cortisol within the body occasionally, because a small amount of stress can sometimes be a positive thing, e.g. a motivator. When cortisol is present for a long period of time constantly, and in high amounts, it can have a very damaging effect on the body and mind. For instance, cortisol easily contributes towards weight gain, especially weight accumulation around the midriff, the common bug-bear of most people who want to shed some pounds.

On a more serious note, cortisol and the stress response can cause a higher risk of heart disease, heart attack, stroke, high blood pressure generally, diabetes, and anxiety and depression. This is not a lifestyle to live voluntarily!

Intermittent fasting can help with stress management because it allows you to achieve your results without denying yourself. For a start, when you're on a low calorie or other restrictive type of diet, you're usually irritable and hungry. This isn't a pleasant life, and it can easily impact on your focus and concentration, your sleep quality, and how you feel generally. As a result, you're not as productive at work, you're making mistakes, and you're becoming stressed because you feel like you're constantly chasing your tail and not making any progress.

Intermittent fasting has been shown to help increase concentration and focus and give more energy. In addition, it helps to improve quality of sleep, and once the body is used to the new way of eating, hunger and cravings are a thing of the past. You're more productive as a result, you're less stressed about making mistakes or not getting anything done, and you'll feel much more 'up' in mood as a result. This helps to banish stress from the get-go and is a fantastic way to ensure that any stressors in your life are easily managed and banished.

Despite the fact that you're actually consuming less calories over the space of a day, you're giving your body a constant source. That might sound incorrect considering the fasting periods, but you're not eating a very small amount and then having to wait until the next day because you've used up all your calories for the day, as is often the case with other low calorie diets - you're free to eat what you want, and that means more satiating foods which are going to keep you fuller for longer. It doesn't matter that they're higher in calories at that point, because you're free to eat what you want in that 'eating window', and the fasting part of it takes care of the rest. You have a constant source of energy for that reason and your body, once it's used to everything, isn't going to be panicking and thinking it's about to starve. That's stressful in enough in itself!

There is a reason that so many people choose the intermittent fasting way these days, and that's because they are fed up of the denial and lack of sustainability with other diets. You shouldn't have to count and add up, weigh out and control everything you eat so carefully. Simply being mindful of what is healthy and what isn't is enough. Intermittent fasting allows you to do this, whilst ensuring that you still lose the weight you want to lose, without the stress and denial you might have been used to in the past.

Chapter 6: Sample Intermittent Fasting Menus

We've talked about the various fasting methods and we've described them in terms of how they work, but what do they look like in practice? This chapter is going to give you a quick snapshot of how you might be able to eat on each method we've covered.

It's hard to give you an exact idea, because there is so much choice with any intermittent fasting method, and no requirement to deny yourself anything. This means that you can easily choose whatever you want (within reason). What we will do however is show you in more real terms, so you can see how each method fits in with a regular lifestyle. Remember, these are not sample menus per se, they are just an example of how you might like to eat - if you want to eat a burger, you can go ahead and do so once day per week; that's what moderation is!

A Sample Week on The 5:2 Diet

A Quick Recap - The 5:2 Diet means that you eat normally for five days of the week and then you fast for two days, although you are allowed to eat 500 calories per day on those 'fasting days'. These two fasting days can't be consecutive, e.g. they need to be spaced apart.

Monday - Normal eating day

Breakfast - Porridge with berries, & a latte
Snack - Banana mid-morning
Lunch - Chicken sandwich with salad, and a yogurt for dessert

Dinner - Lasagne and salad, and a low-fat chocolate mousse for dessert

Tuesday - Fasting day

Breakfast - Greek yogurt with sultanas and almonds (94 calories)
Lunch - Crushed new potatoes with bamboo shoots and boiled egg (186 calories)
Dinner - Chinese vegetable chow Mein (170 calories)
Snack - Two satsumas (50 calories)

Wednesday - Normal eating day

Breakfast - Boiled egg and two slices of toast, cup of coffee
Snack - Yogurt and some berries
Lunch - Tuna pasta salad
Dinner - Jacket potato with whatever topping you like

Thursday - Normal eating day

Breakfast - Fried egg and bacon, cooked with low fat cooking spray, and a coffee
Lunch - Tomato soup and a small bread roll
Snack - An apple and two satsumas
Dinner - Two slices of pizza and salad

Friday - Fasting day

Breakfast - Spinach omelette made with two eggs (94 calories)
Lunch - Chicken miso soup (126 calories)
Dinner - Moroccan root tagging with a side of couscous (230 calories)
Snack - Two satsumas (50 calories)

Saturday - Normal eating day

Breakfast - Grilled bacon roll and coffee
Snack - Yogurt and banana
Lunch - Tuna and pasta salad
Dinner - It's the weekend and you can eat out and have whatever you want!

Sunday - Normal eating day

Breakfast - Grilled bacon and fried eggs with toast
Snack - An apple and satsuma
Lunch - Sunday roast with meat, potatoes, vegetables, gravy, etc.
Dinner - Cold meat sandwich with salad

A Sample Week on The 16:8 Diet

A Quick Recap - The 16:8 diet means that you eat freely for eight hours and you fast for the rest. You can choose your specific eating window and fasting window, but the 16 hours need to be consecutive. You can also incorporate your sleeping hours into these fasting hours.

Because this diet has a lot of scope, i.e. you choose when you fast and when you don't, we'll assume that you've chosen a 12pm until 8pm eating window, with fasting for the rest.

Monday

Begin eating at 12pm - Meal 1 - Two boiled eggs with two slices of toast, and a glass of orange juice

Snack - Coffee and a slice of fruit loaf
Meal 2 - Jacket potato and salad with a topping of your choice
Meal 3 - Warm chicken baguette and salad
Snack - Low fat chocolate mousse

Finish eating at 8pm. During fasting hours consume water, and unsweetened, black tea and coffee to stay hydrated.

Tuesday

Begin eating at 12pm - Meal 1 - Porridge oats with berries and a coffee
Snack - Fruit salad
Meal 2 - Tuna pasta salad
Meal 3 - Spaghetti Bolognese
Snack - Yogurt

Finish eating at 8pm. During fasting hours consume water, and unsweetened, black tea and coffee to stay hydrated.

Wednesday

Begin eating at 12pm - Meal 1 - Grilled cheese sandwich and orange juice
Snack - Fruit salad
Meal 2 - Chicken salad and couscous
Meal 3 - Salmon and grilled vegetables
Snack - Slice of fruit cake

Finish eating at 8pm. During fasting hours consume water, and unsweetened, black tea and coffee to stay hydrated.

Thursday

Begin eating at 12pm - Meal 1 - Two slices of toast with jam and a coffee
Snack - Banana
Meal 2 - A bowl of tomato soup with one bread roll
Meal 3 - Chicken and potato stew
Snack - Yogurt

Finish eating at 8pm. During fasting hours consume water, and unsweetened, black tea and coffee to stay hydrated.

Friday

Begin eating at 12pm - Meal 1 - Grilled bacon and mushroom roll with a coffee
Snack - Pineapple slices
Meal 2 - Spicy chicken wrap and yogurt for dessert
Meal 3 - Spaghetti carbonara
Snack - Fruit salad

Finish eating at 8pm. During fasting hours consume water, and unsweetened, black tea and coffee to stay hydrated.

Saturday

Begin eating at 12pm - Meal 1 - Mashed avocado on toast with a coffee
Snack - Slice of fruit loaf
Meal 2 - It's the weekend! You can eat out for lunch and enjoy your food of choice
Meal 3 - Salad of your choice
Snack - Fruit salad

Finish eating at 8pm. During fasting hours consume water, and unsweetened, black tea and coffee to stay hydrated.

Sunday

Begin eating at 12pm - Meal 1 - Granola and yogurt
Snack - And apple and satsuma
Meal 2 - Two slices of toast with whatever topping you like
Meal 3 - Sunday roast with potatoes, vegetables, meat, Yorkshire pudding, gravy etc.
Snack - Low fat chocolate mousse

Finish eating at 8pm. During fasting hours consume water, and unsweetened, black tea and coffee to stay hydrated.

A Sample Week on The 800 Fast Diet

A Quick Recap - This is the newest kid on the dieting block and it has a stage of eating 800 calories for day for two weeks, before switching to the 5:2 Diet as above, with the difference that you need to eat your two fasting day meals within a 10-hour window and you can have 800 calories per day on those days, rather than the regular 500.

For the purposes of this plan, let's look at a week on the first phase, e.g. consuming 800 calories for per day. After the two weeks, switch to the 5:2 design. These recipes are quite regularly used, and can be found online.

Monday

Breakfast - Scrambled eggs
Lunch - Fennel, citrus and asparagus salad
Dinner - Pork loin wrapped in prosciutto and rice

Tuesday

Breakfast - Yogurt and berries
Lunch - Humus and carrot/celery sticks
Dinner - Spicy crab casserole

Wednesday

Breakfast - Berry smoothie with banana
Lunch - Fruit salad
Dinner - Ceviche with smoked salmon

Thursday

Breakfast - Smoked salmon and avocado
Lunch - Fruit salad
Dinner - Sausage and vegetable tray bake

Friday

Breakfast - Yogurt and berries
Lunch - Apple beetroot and bean soup
Dinner - Fish pie with topping made of celeriac

Saturday

Breakfast - Green smoothie
Lunch - Mustard and crab lettuce wraps
Dinner - White bean mash and grilled chicken

Sunday

Breakfast - Fruit salad
Lunch - Yogurt with a handful of berries and chia seeds
Dinner - Pork, apple and shallot tray bake

A Sample Week on The Warrior Diet

A Quick Recap - The Warrior Diet is one which will test your warrior spirit and actually means you need to fast (with a very low intake of certain products) for 20 hours of the day and then consume whatever you want for the remaining hours, at night. For those evening hours, you are actually encouraged to binge eat, in order to get a good amount of sustenance, but it's not a great idea to binge on unhealthy produce, to avoid stomach aches.

This sample will assume the day begins at 12am, and therefore you are unable to eat properly from 12am until 8pm in the evening. Some of that you will be sleeping, but the remaining hours of the day require you to eat very little else. Be sure to get plenty of water for hydration.

We won't give you a specific eating plan for this diet as it is so difficult to break down, but highlight how it works a little more clearly instead.

Monday to Sunday

From 12am until 8pm - 2 hard boiled eggs, a handful of raw vegetables and fresh fruits, a yogurt. Drink plenty of water.

8pm until 12am - You can either have one large meal, or two smaller ones, and then snack until the 12am hour arrives, when you then stop. It's a good idea to ensure that you get:

- Carbs
- Protein
- Calcium
- Plenty of vegetables and fruit content

Avoid eating heavy foods, e.g. fast food pizzas, burgers, chips, and instead go for the slow release, healthy options, such as porridge, brown bread, brown pasta, whole-grains etc.

It is extremely difficult to give you an eating plan for this diet, but simply advise you to use common sense during your 4-hour window. There is no limit on calorie intake, but remember that if you overload your stomach, you're going to feel terrible and might have a few undesirable side effects.

A Sample Week Alternate Day Fasting Method

A Quick Recap - As the name suggests, the alternate day fasting method means you eat normally one day and then fast the next. You can change this up and eat a low-calorie intake of 500 if you want to on the fasting days. For the purposes of this meal plan, we'll assume that you're going for the normal eating pattern, and then a 500-calorie day option. Make sure that you drink plenty of water and unsweetened black tea and coffee throughout the day, to ensure you stay hydrated, fasting or not.

Monday - Normal eating day

Breakfast - Scrambled egg on toast with a glass of orange juice
Snack - Fruit salad
Lunch - Chicken wrap with yogurt and coffee
Dinner - Lasagne

Tuesday - Fasting/low calorie day

Breakfast - Two Ryvita crackers and Marmite spread
Lunch - Tomato soup
Dinner - Grilled chicken and vegetables

Wednesday - Normal eating day

Breakfast - Grilled cheese sandwich (low calorie cheese)
Snack - An apple and satsuma
Lunch - Tuna pasta salad
Dinner - Grilled chicken and potatoes in the oven

Thursday - Fasting/low calorie day

Breakfast - Low fat yogurt and chopped up fruit, e.g. apricots
Snack - Apple
Lunch - Broccoli and stilton soup
Dinner - Roasted ratatouille

Friday - Normal eating day

Breakfast - Grilled bacon roll and coffee
Snack - Banana
Lunch - Jacket potato and chilli
Dinner - Fish and boiled potatoes

Saturday - Fasting/low calorie days

Breakfast - Cinnamon toast
Snack - Two satsumas
Lunch - Mushroom soup
Dinner - Spicy tomato pasta

Sunday - Normal eating day

Breakfast - Fried egg (with low fat cooking spray) with mushrooms, grilled tomato and toast
Snack - An apple
Lunch - Sunday roast with potatoes, meat, gravy, vegetables, and Yorkshire pudding
Dinner - Cold meat sandwich and salad

As you can see, these sample weeks show you that intermittent fasting, no matter which option you go for, certainly doesn't leave you hungry! Perhaps the word 'fasting' is misleading, because there is no point where you are starving at all! Remember, fasting and starving are two very different things. The only 'on the fence' options is the Warrior Diet, which includes long periods of not eating very much at all, followed by a short period of eating anything you like. It's very likely that this period is going to mean you binge on everything you crave, and that is going to lead to possible stomach disturbances, and in some cases, you might even put weight on, depending on how much you actually eat!

Chapter 7: Dos & Don'ts of Intermittent Fasting

We're almost at the end of our journey into the intermittent fasting world, and by now you should be feeling positive and uplifted about the options in front of you. Provided you make the right choice and decide upon a method which really suits your needs and your lifestyle, you won't notice a huge difference in your day to day routine. The only difference you will notice is the pounds dropping off and you feeling far better in yourself!

Of course, there are a few dos and don'ts we need to talk about, because this is a change in your lifestyle pattern and as a result you need to be aware of possible side effects, things to be on the lookout for, and what you should and shouldn't do. This chapter is going to cover all of those things. First things first, let's talk about what the medical world think about intermittent fasting.

The Medical Take on Intermittent Fasting

There is no specific concern about intermittent fasting per se, however some studies do state that women may find it harder to have an intermittent fasting lifestyle than men. This is all down to hormones and the way they fluctuate.

Women's bodies are extremely sensitive to changes in calorie intake, and the slightest tip of the scales can mean that hormones are thrown out of whack. When this happens, a few side effects occur, some mild, some moderate, and some serious. For this reason, modified versions of intermittent fasting methods are best. For instance, the alternate day method isn't the greatest for a woman when you literally eat what you want for one day and then fast completely for another, with the cycle continuing in that way. That is why the modified version of eating a low intake of 500 calories and then eating what you want cycle was implemented. Whilst 500 calories is still low, it isn't dangerous on an alternate day pattern. It would however become dangerous over a longer period of sustained time.

Most women know when their hormones are out of balance, because you simply feel not yourself. You might be extremely agitated for no real reason, you might feel overly emotional, headachy, and have stomach upsets. These are all symptoms of PMS, but these also mirror the symptoms of hormones not being in balance. Feeling lethargic and completely lacking in energy is another.

What you certainly should be on the lookout for is any sign that your menstrual periods are changing. This could mean that your intermittent fasting routine is not the best one for you and is causing your hormonal levels to be out of balance. This could mean that periods either stop altogether, or become irregular, light or heavier. In this case, speak to your doctor and consider either stopping intermittent fasting altogether, or simply change your method to something which is less drastic on your body. The Warrior Diet is one which isn't the greatest for women, that's for sure, and causes huge ups and downs with sugar levels, as well as general hormones, which are so closely linked.

Obviously, if you have any health concerns or you're on any medications then you should speak to your doctor before you being with intermittent fasting anyway. We mentioned this earlier in the book and it's something we need to reiterate again. The medical opinion of intermittent fasting is that it is generally safe and very effective when done correctly, but rules need to be followed and symptoms should be monitored. It's also very important to make sure that you get plenty of hydration throughout the day, be it water or unsweetened black tea or black coffee. Basically, any beverage which contains no calories is fine and encouraged.

The Do's of Intermittent Fasting

Do Get Yourself Checked Out Before You Begin Intermittent Fasting

If you have any type of health concern, you're on any medications, you're breastfeeding, or you have any type of issue with your overall health and wellbeing, get yourself checked out with your doctor. However, even if you consider yourself to be fighting fit, it doesn't hurt to have a quick check over with your doctor, a health MOT of sorts, before you begin with your fasting endeavours.

Do Choose a Method Which Fits Into Your Regular Lifestyle

There is an intermittent fasting method for everyone so you will easily be able to fit the right one into your regular lifestyle. This means if you have a hobby which you enjoy every week, perhaps even a wine tasting evening you do every couple of weeks, or a weekly night out with your friends at a restaurant you can factor this into your diet, on one of the days when you're able to eat freely. In this case, you would simply make wise choices, rather than not being able to do go out at all.

Do Weigh up The Pros And Cons of Each Method

Be sure to really read through all the methods before you and check the pros and cons. Don't just go with the most popular, because the most popular might not be the ideal choice for you. We're all individuals at the end of the day and you need to think as you and you alone. By know the pros and cons of each method you are free to make the right decision, and a well-informed decision too.

Do Clear Out Your Kitchen in Preparation
It's a great idea to have a kitchen clear out before you begin. This will get rid of any added temptations and make sure that you do make healthy choices, even though you're not restricted per se. Remember, 'eat what you want' doesn't literally mean go down to the local pizza place and have a full pizza to yourself - it means eat the things you like in moderation! Having a kitchen stocked with unhealthy snacks means you're far more likely to reach for something sugar or fat laden, rather than something healthier.

Do Remember Your Reason For Starting
We mentioned earlier on about knowing why you're actually doing the intermittent fasting route in the first place. You're going to have times, especially at the start, when your body isn't quite sure what's happening yet and needs a little time to adjust. During this period, you might have side effects or hunger that is hard to deal with. When you know your reason and you really believe in it, you can minimise any problems and jump over that first challenging hurdle.

Do Incorporate Exercise Into Your Routine
Exercise is great for your overall health and wellbeing, including for your mental health and mood too. By incorporating exercise into your routine, you'll boost your

weight loss efforts and give your overall health a push in the right direction. Find a sport or activity you enjoy and go for it. You could also look to make changes into your routine, e.g. walking to work rather than driving or going on the bus, taking the stairs rather than the elevator, and going for a stroll during your lunch hour. These changes will all add up!

Do Think About Vitamin Supplements
It might be a good idea to have a chat with your doctor about any vitamin supplements you should be taking. When you change your eating habits, it is sometimes the case that you lack certain vitamins and minerals. When this goes on for a long period of time, you begin to notice symptoms of that deficiency and these can sometimes be damaging. By taking appropriate supplements, you can avoid this issue. Again, always chat to your doctor before you begin taking any type of vitamin supplementation.

Do Enlist The Help of Friends And Family
Tell your friends and family what you're doing and why, and have their help to get you through any difficult times. You could even ask if they want to do it with you - having a buddy in the intermittent fasting world is sometimes a great motivator to carry on!

The Don'ts of Intermittent Fasting

Don't Forget to Inform Your Doctor
We've mentioned this a few times but it's so super-important that we need to mention it at least once more! Remember to inform your doctor whenever you make any huge changes to your diet and lifestyle. Just a quick chat is all it will take to make sure that you're fit and healthy for fasting of any kind and avoid any problems

which may turn out to be serious in the future. Even if you think you're healthy, a quick MOT is a good idea. Sometimes we don't realise we have a specific problem or condition until someone else highlights it, perhaps through a blood test, or simply by chatting about a symptom that you had no idea was of significance.

Don't Overload Your Stomach When You Are Allowed to Eat

At first especially, it's likely that when you are able to eat, you might overload your stomach by eating anything and everything. It's also likely that you'll grab high fat and high sugar choices which will leave you feeling stomach achy and have your blood sugar crashing a short while later. You'll no doubt make this mistake at least once when you begin, but you'll also quickly learn that it's not a good idea! Instead, stick with slow release, healthy choices, and pace yourself as much as you can. If you can drip feed your stomach the things it needs, it's less likely to throw disturbances your way, basically stamping its metaphorical feet in protest! Pace yourself.

Don't Assume You Can Eat Fast Food Whenever The Method Says 'No Limits'

Intermittent fasting is so popular, but also because people mistakenly think that 'eat what you want' means literally eat pizzas, burgers, takeaways in abundance. If you're looking for that type of diet or eating routine, you're going to be searching forever more. These types of foods simply aren't healthy when eating in large amounts or on a regular basis. What you can do however, as part of the intermittent fasting routine, is have a takeaway of this kind in moderation. For instance, you could have a couple of slices of pizza one night in the week. You'll find that you enjoy it far more because you're not denying yourself, but you're also not having it too often, to the point where it's no longer special.

Even though intermittent fasting doesn't force you to deny yourself anything, you should still make healthy food choices for your overall wellbeing. If you binge on calories during your eating period, it doesn't matter that you're fasting for a length of time afterwards, because you've still amassed too many calories. The number of calories in fast food can be startling!

Don't Forget to Listen to Your Body

Always listen to your body and never push your limits beyond what feels comfortable. If the method you choose doesn't suit you, your body will tell you. If you feel unwell when doing any intermittent fasting method, stop and speak to your doctor. If you notice unpleasant side effects which don't seem to be improving, again, stop and speak to your doctor. In most cases, it's simply that you chose the wrong option for you and you need to seek out a better one, which suits your body and doesn't cause unpleasant side effects. Remember, we're all different and one size never fits all. Listen to your body and follow its guidance, it knows the way.

Don't Forget to Drink Plenty of Water

Even when you are in your fasting or low calorie periods, you need to stay hydrated. This is one of the most important steps of intermittent fasting. The word fasting pertains to food and calorie intake, it doesn't pertain to calorie-free liquids, which your body needs regardless. If you cut out water, you're going to become ill quite quickly.

What you can do is drink as much water as you like when you're on your low-calorie times or when you're fasting, and you can also enjoy unsweetened black tea or coffee also. Any type of beverage which has no calories at all can be enjoyed, and it is encouraged that you do so, to ensure you do not fall into the realms of dehydration. A good way to remind yourself to drink is to keep a bottle of water by your bed, in your car, in your bag, and by your desk.

You'll probably also come to realise that a lot of the time when you think you're hungry, you're really not. It's more likely that you're either bored, or even more likely, you're thirsty. In this case, a drink of water can be enough to take the edge off what you consider to be hungry, and leave you satiated in the way you need.

Don't Allow Stress to Become an Issue
When you first start an intermittent fasting method of any kind, it's possible that you'll get a little stressed out with it. The reason is because it's a change and as humans we don't really like change too much. Our bodies also don't like change and this can cause side effects. Remember, the transitional period might be a little difficult, with a few unwanted side effects, but it should not be tortuous and it should not be impossible. Do not allow yourself to become stressed out as this is going to make things worse, by increasing the amount of cortisol (stress hormone) you have winging its way around your body. When cortisol amounts are high, you're more likely to hit a weight loss plateau or actually gain it, regardless of your efforts.

The intermittent fasting method you choose should also not cause you undue stress. You should pick a method that you understand freely and that doesn't cause you any problems within your lifestyle. Intermittent fasting is supposed to positively affect and compliment your life, and not affect it in a negative way.

Final Thoughts

The dos and don'ts of intermittent fasting aren't difficult to follow or understand. You simply need to choose the right option for you and listen to your body. If you notice something which you feel just isn't quite right, you should pay attention to that sign and do something about it. Changing your intermittent fasting method can sometimes be all it takes to work things out and allow you to continue onwards, and therefore grab the benefits.

The biggest 'do' to remember is to hydrate your body at all times. This will give you a clearer focus, probably get rid of hunger in many cases, and also ensure that you don't suffer from dehydration effects, such as headaches and shakiness. Dehydration is not something to voluntarily bring on, so make sure you stay hydrated, even when you're supposed to be fasting - drinks don't always have calories in them, and you need to make these a priority.

Conclusion

And there we have it! We've reached the end of our book about intermittent fasting and you now know everything there is to know about losing weight, detoxing, cleansing your body, and boosting your concentration levels.

Intermittent fasting is very popular in the health and wellness world for a good reason. When followed correctly, and when there are no contraindications, your method of choice will guide you towards your weight loss goals, but it will also bring many other health and wellness benefits that you probably never even dreamed could come your way.

The concept of fasting has been around for centuries, and it has never caused harm when it is understood and followed correctly. Remember, there is a very real difference between fasting and starvation. You are choosing to abstain from food for a specific length of time when fasting, but you are also giving the intention to eat properly during the other hours of the day. When you are starving yourself, you have no intention to eat, and therefore you only have the intention to do sometimes irreversible damage to your mind and body. The difference is huge, so never become worried by hearing the word 'fasting'.

Humans have been fasting for centuries for various different reasons, and many religions also incorporate periods of fasting in order to bring the person greater clarity of mind. The benefits are certainly very impressive, and provide you choose the right intermittent fasting method based on you as an individual, you'll be able to follow this new pattern of eating for a long period of time.

You see, the difference between intermittent fasting and regular diets, especially fad diets, is that it isn't a diet at all. Intermittent fasting is a routine, a new lifestyle, and it is something which is designed to be sustainable over the long-term. Of course, when you no longer want to lose weight and you have reached your target, you need to look at your calorie intake and make sure that you hit a maintenance level, possibly by increasing your calorie intake over the course of a day. For the initial phase however, e.g. when you want to lose weight, intermittent fasting is a sure-fire way to hit your targets, with a lot less stress and hassle then regular so-called diets.

There is nothing enjoyable about restricting your calorie intake to low amounts over a long period of time. Life is far too short to be miserable! There are far too many delicious foods out there which are begging to be tried, and if you deny yourself the chance, in the end you will rebel against the whole idea and give in. At that time, you'll feel like you've failed, and your confidence will drop to new lows.

By choosing intermittent fasting, you're breaking the cycle of dietary failures int he past, and you're committing to success. You're also putting your health and wellness first, provided you check things out with your doctor before you begin. From there, choosing the right method for you is the next step. Changes can be made with no problems if you make the wrong decision, but being armed with all the information you need from the get-go will ensure that you don't make an incorrect decision at all, and you can simply continue onwards from the start and reach your goals much faster as a result.

All that is really left for us to say now is good luck! We hope that you have found the information contained within this book helpful and motivating, and we hope that by adopting an intermittent fasting lifestyle, you will reach your goals and grab the health benefits which work alongside a period of fasting and eating on a daily basis.

By listening to your body and understanding what it needs versus what it wants, you'll learn a lot, but you'll also notice your confidence soaring too. As you drop those pounds, you feel lighter on your feet, you feel less fuzzy in your mind, and the future looks very bright indeed!

Please see other Titles from

ARYLA PUBLISHING

Children's Books
The Body Goo Series
The Billy Series
The Ruby Series
Emergency Service Series
Love Bugs & Animals Series

Adult Books
Self Help Books
Diet and Wellbeing
Comedy Books

FOR ALL
Coloring Books

Other Publications

Giving Up Sugar –
By Sharon Kingsley (Self Help)

You love sweets, and you think that nothing in this world could dissuade you from eating them. But what about the fact that sugar is also called "sweet poison"? And did you know it can destroy your body, just like one of the zombies in the popular TV series "The Walking Dead"? Those horrible creatures feast on human internal organs as if they were succulent dishes. Ew, That's what accumulated sugar does to your internal organs, as well.

Excessive sugar obliterates your organs until nothing is left to perform their physiologic functions. In case you're one of the few, who haven't seen this TV series, then you may want to watch to see how this gory process takes place. If you're already convinced of the importance of eliminating sugar in your diet, read on, and learn how you can overcome it.

Diet Fads

By Sharon Kingsley (Health & Wellbeing)

There are times in life when we want to look our very best. Of course, you might want to look your very best most of the time, but there are general occasions when this is more important than ever before. We're talking about events such as weddings (either yours or someone else's), vacations, a big party looming on the horizon, that kind of thing.

These types of events require us not only to have our hair done perfectly, make up contoured to perfection, nails immaculate, and eyebrows tweezed to within an inch of their lives, but they also require us to look our slimmest too.

Whether this is wrong or right, it's the truth of the matter. If you're getting married, you want to get into that dress, or into that tuxedo, without feeling extra pounds spilling over the top. If you're heading off on vacation, you want to head to the beach without feeling self-conscious. If you're about to attend a big party or function, you want people to be talking about how fantastic you look, not how you've gained a few pounds.

Whether you're male or female, everyone wants to hit that happy weight. Your happy weight is completely personal to you; it doesn't need to be skinny, it doesn't need to be curvy, it's a weight at which your body settles into a natural plateau, where you can look your best, feel fantastic, and wear whatever you want.

Anxiety: Dealing With Anxiety & Panic Attacks –
By Fiona Welsh (Self Help)

Do you regularly feel like you are always worrying about something? Do you often feel fearful? Do you wake up with a sense of dread a lot of the time? Do you feel fine one minute and then you start overthinking, and your mind turns into a hamster wheel of 'what if' situations and scenarios? Do you feel generally uneasy a lot of the time, and you can't really pinpoint a reason why?

If you are nodding your head to most of the above then it could very well be that you are suffering from an anxiety disorder.

Anxiety is more common than you might even think. It is thought that 1 in every 13 people will suffer from an anxiety disorder at some stage in their lives, and this equates to around 7.3% of the world's population. The statistics are startling, and that makes anxiety the most common mental disorder in the spectrum.

If you're feeling like you might have a problem with anxiety, these statistics should give you a little hope – you're not alone, you're not going crazy, the world isn't the dark place that you might be led to believe; there is help at hand.

The Truth About Getting Old –
By Tyler Moses (Comedy)

Congratulations and welcome to the over 40s club! You have worked hard to get to this pinnacle point in life, so let's take a moment to celebrate being over 40 and everything that comes with it. Your body has been through a lot in order to get you over the hill, and your 40s is when some of your parts may start to, well, retire. During your time in the old person club, your body will experience new and not-so-exciting changes around every corner (even though we take corners slowly now as to avoid obstacles that may knock us off balance). Grab your Biotene and a large supply of antacids and sit back on your heating pad as we journey into the life of being over 40.

Julia's Dilemma –
By Lyndsey Carter (Romantic Comedy)

Julia sighed as she stepped onto the escalator. As it moved and took her up, she sighed again. Another boring day and another crammed ride home on a smelly train with no seats. She longed for some excitement, something to shake things up. She was sick of the same old, same old.

Julie boarded the train, already knowing as she craned her neck to scan each corner that there would not be any seats open. Instead, she settled for a hand-hold on the pole near the back wall. But her surroundings ceased to bother her as she stared off into the distance and let her thoughts roam. She looked at the houses she passed and imagined what type of people lived there. The train line ran at the back of the houses giving Julie a view of the garden. Some gardens had washing hanging up; others had kids' toys. Some gardens were overgrown like a mini jungle. It was a little daydream game Julia liked to play when she didn't have a book or paper to read. Soon the passing gardens and motion of the train made her eyes heavy.

Julia fought to keep her eyes open, scared that she would miss her stop. Even after six years of riding the same train back and forth to work, she was still afraid that she would fall asleep and ride until the train reached the end of the line.

We also have a selection of Adult Coloring Books to help relax pass the time and de-stress.
Beautiful Illustrations and puzzles for your entertainment

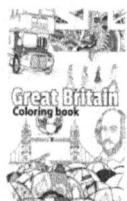

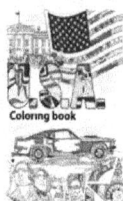

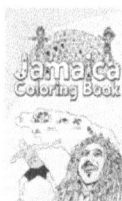

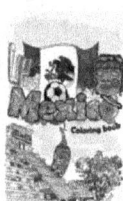

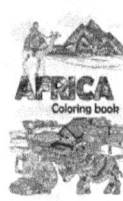

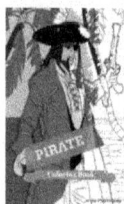

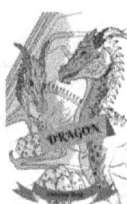

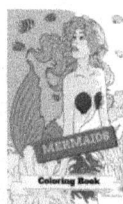

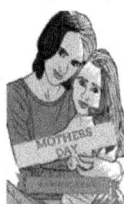

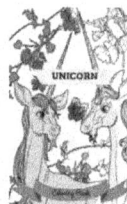

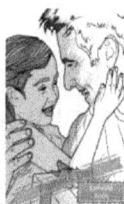

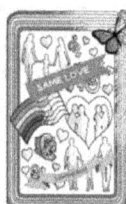

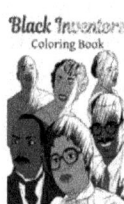

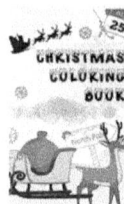

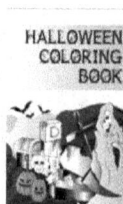

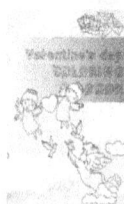

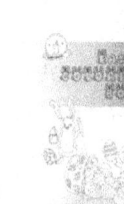